the
herbal
doula

the
herbal
doula

plant medicine for fertility, community care, and birthwork

marie white

North Atlantic Books
Huichin, unceded Ohlone land
Berkeley, California

Published by
North Atlantic Books
Huichin, unceded Ohlone land
Berkeley, California

Cover photo © Ivelin Denev via Getty Images
Cover design by Jess Morphew
Book design by Happenstance Type-O-Rama

Printed in the United States of America

The Herbal Doula: Plant Medicine for Fertility, Community Care, and Birthwork is sponsored and published by North Atlantic Books, an educational nonprofit based in the unceded Ohlone land Huichin (Berkeley, CA) that collaborates with partners to develop cross-cultural perspectives; nurture holistic views of art, science, the humanities, and healing; and seed personal and global transformation by publishing work on the relationship of body, spirit, and nature.

North Atlantic Books's publications are distributed to the US trade and internationally by Penguin Random House Publisher Services. For further information, visit our website at www.northatlanticbooks.com.

Library of Congress Cataloging-in-Publication Data
Names: White, Marie, 1991- author.
Title: The herbal doula : plant medicine for fertility, community care, and birthwork / Marie White.
Description: Berkeley, California : North Atlantic Books, [2024] | Includes bibliographical references and index.
Identifiers: LCCN 2024000923 (print) | LCCN 2024000924 (ebook) | ISBN 9781623179427 (trade paperback) | ISBN 9781623179434 (ebook) | ISBN 9781623179434 (ebook)
Subjects: LCSH: Herbal contraceptives. | Herbs--Therapeutic use. | Prenatal care. | Postnatal care.
Classification: LCC RG137.45 .W45 2024 (print) | LCC RG137.45 (ebook) | DDC 613.9/4--dc23/eng/20240411
LC record available at https://lccn.loc.gov/2024000923
LC ebook record available at https://lccn.loc.gov/2024000924.

1 2 3 4 5 6 7 8 9 KPC 28 27 26 25 24

This book includes recycled material and material from well-managed forests. North Atlantic Books is committed to the protection of our environment. We print on recycled paper whenever possible and partner with printers who strive to use environmentally responsible practices.

Contents

Introduction
About *The Herbal Doula*

Pregnancy and birth are at once ordinary and transformative. Every day and across cultures, people become pregnant and give birth. But when it happens to you, there's nothing ordinary or mundane about it. Throughout time, doulas have been supporting folks along the conception, pregnancy, birth, and postpartum journey. Doulas are partners and allies present to support and nurture before, during, and beyond birth.

The presence of a doula during pregnancy and birth brings many therapeutic benefits. For instance, pregnant people and their partners report happier memories of their delivery when they're supported by a doula. It's not surprising that care and support would improve birth outcomes. But doulas can help with so much more than pregnancy and birth. Their care work is also needed while trying to conceive and when facing infertility, during postpartum recovery, and through pregnancy loss like miscarriage or abortion. Yes, if you're thinking that everyone needs a doula on their whole reproductive journey, you're right! And this is partly what *The Herbal Doula* book seeks to offer you.

If you're pregnant or planning to become pregnant, this book will offer you guidance and support in being your own budding fertility, conception, and pregnancy doula. It will guide you along tips and wisdom for birth and postpartum and caring for yourself and your baby with the help of medicinal herbs. And if you have a doula—or doulas—on your care team (and I hope you do!), this book will serve as a handy companion you can refer to over and over. You'll find within these pages trusted information on plant medicine and reproductive wellness.

The Herbal Doula is also meant as a guide and herbal reference for birthworkers, full spectrum doulas and midwives, fertility coaches, herbalists, and folks working in the pregnancy and birth realm who are curious about blending medicinal herbs with birthwork and advocacy. Medicinal herbs are beneficial, therapeutic, safe, and effective additions to your work and practice. Your community will benefit from you learning about plant medicine as it relates to fertility and pregnancy. Many of your friends and clients are already using herbs, and they will count on you for advice and herbal guidance.

My goal is to offer you a reliable, accessible, and engaging guide you can return to again and again. I will introduce you to the wisdom of plants in a way that is rooted in daily practice and community care, while exploring medicinal home-based remedies. As an herbal practitioner, I have a commitment to empowering folks to engage with their health and wellness from an open and inclusive way. In *The Herbal Doula,* you will learn everything you need to know to work with healing herbs with confidence and trust as you support your own or others' reproductive journeys.

I've been working and playing with herbs as an herbalist for about fifteen years now. I grow medicinal herbs in our regenerative gardens, make herbal remedies and medicine from scratch, teach herbal students, and offer herbal consultations. To accompany people along their pregnancies and births is a real joy and privilege. Of course, this support includes infertility, miscarriages, and abortions, all of which are more common than you might think, and which strongly benefit from herbal support and doula care too.

I've coached clients along as they explore fertility challenges like infertility and go through fertility treatments. I've created herbal protocols for common pregnancy conditions as well as for birth support.

Some births have been easier for people while other births were harder. Some folks experience postpartum depression while others don't. The whole process is so personal and varied, but whatever happens, one thing is certain: Herbs can help.

You don't have to be a trained doula or herbalist to learn from *The Herbal Doula.* Anyone interested in care and nurturing, fertility and pregnancy, birth and postpartum, and plant medicine is invited and welcomed to dive deep into this emergent and nourishing work and practice. Doula herbalism embraces the recognition that "well-resourced and supported families create thriving communities," in the words of the kind folks at Partum Gardens in Portland, Oregon, a community care collective that supports parents and children through weekly garden gatherings. To "care for birthing bodies and their families" is a seed we can plant together, tending to our healing herbs, our community, our clients, and ourselves.

Pregnancy and birth are ordinary processes; they are also precious, tender, and life-changing. Caring for those who experience pregnancy and give birth is both essential and radical. It has the potential to alter lives and relationships and communities. My hope is that you find in this book inspiration and a wholehearted desire to ally yourself with plants in this process. I'm honored to be your guide along the way.

How to Use This Book

The guide you hold in your hands was created as a reference manual for blending herbal medicine and reproductive wellness. The framework of *The Herbal Doula* is to focus on safe, gentle, and accessible herbs while approaching your reproductive journey from a radically inclusive and welcoming lens. As such, it is written in a way that seeks to be open to various ways of becoming pregnant and all safe birthing choices that are right for you and your child, whether you choose to breastfeed or not, and everything that can happen in between.

It has become popular to use divisive and binary language—like natural versus unnatural, or alternative versus conventional, for example.

You won't find that in this book. The care strategies laid out in *The Herbal Doula* are inclined toward collaborative medicine and complementary herbal therapies. It equips you to partner with many layers of care professionals and to ally yourself with their ways along with your chosen herbal practices, be it in a clinic, a hospital, or at home. The herbal framework laid out in these pages is rooted in home-based practices, the types of which can be interwoven with food traditions and home life.

I also have a commitment to body neutrality in my herbal practice, which means that I rely on a "Health at Every Size" approach to weight and health. I don't use body mass index (BMI), which is a flawed metric anyway, or body weight as a measure of health and fertility or as any measure of reproductive ability and capacity to become pregnant, to go through in vitro fertilization (IVF), to give birth, to adopt, or to raise children.

Fat people experience too many hurdles on their journey to pregnancy and birth, such as being told by medical professionals, "You just need to lose weight" (to borrow a phrase from fat activist and author Aubrey Gordon)[1] or other statements or measures that display anti-fat bias. Examples of weight-based discrimination in the pregnancy realm have included some IVF clinics across North America refusing to serve fat patients, as well as certain adoption agencies who won't allow fat adoptive parents to complete the adoption process. But people of all sizes and body shapes can get pregnant, give birth, be parents, care for children, and use herbs for support along the way.

Other commitments integral to the practice of doula herbalism laid out in these pages include antiracism. Acknowledging and fighting racism are essential to birthwork because Black, Indigenous, and people of color (BIPOC) folks continue to experience substandard medical care due to the impacts of widespread systemic racism. Where I live and work, in North America, these structural inequalities show up in the pregnancy, birth, and postpartum realm through a higher maternal and child mortality rate in Black, Hispanic, and Indigenous folks when compared with their white counterparts.

Other examples of the impacts of racism in the field of reproductive health include a higher rate of polycystic ovary syndrome (PCOS) in Hispanic and South Asian people, as well as a higher risk of preterm birth in Black and Indigenous folks compared with white people. If you care about the health of pregnant and birthing people, challenging systemic racism by providing accessible and equal health care is an important facet of your work.

Care for queer families is also central to the practice of doula herbalism. There are so many ways to become a parent, and so many possible iterations of family. What's more, medicinal herbs have a strong tradition of use among the queer and trans communities. As Toi Scott wrote in *Queering Herbalism,* "Queer and transgender folks were often healers in their societies," and they have been involved in the healing of their communities throughout generations.[2]

People experience pregnancy and birth differently based on social, cultural, economic, and other intersectional factors. Social determinants of health can and should be taken into consideration when working with herbs and when choosing which types of herbal remedies, recipes, and rituals are best suited to you and your own circumstances and needs. Plant medicine is accessible and intuitive, and it will look different for different folks.

Before we dive deeper into *The Herbal Doula* and its practices, let's touch on earth care and sustainability. Medicinal herbs are living organisms that require specific environments in which to grow and thrive. Protecting biodiversity, supporting pollinators like native bees and migratory birds, and prioritizing the use of herbs sourced from local organic, biodynamic, or regenerative gardens when possible will help make your herbal practice sustainable and restorative for generations to come.

Because we live in times of environmental upheaval, you'll find tips and instructions on herbal medicine for such modern concerns as excessive heat and exposure to wildfire smoke. Heat and smoke are especially dangerous for pregnant folks as well as young children. With the compounded impacts of climate change, high temperatures and wildfires are only becoming more likely. Thankfully, medicinal herbs have a lot to offer in terms of remedy and comfort.

Let's talk about the book. Chapters in *The Herbal Doula* are divided by reproductive events, starting with fertility and trying to conceive. The chapters then progress in order from miscarriage and abortion, pregnancy and birth, and postpartum and breastfeeding to baby and child care. A final section also explores recommended herbs and herbal practices for doulas and birthworkers.

A set of herbs is discussed in each chapter, with information specifically tailored to that reproductive event. You will notice that some of the same herbs come up over and over from one chapter to the next. This is normal; in each chapter, you'll learn a new facet of the same herbs. At the end of the book, you'll find a doula herbalism Materia Medica that finally puts it all together and compiles a full herb profile for you to easily refer to.

These herbs are your special allies in the reproductive realm. They're safe, accessible, and multipurpose throughout your experience of pregnancy, birth, postpartum, and beyond. The idea isn't to use all these herbs, but rather to find the ones within the herbs listed that have the most affinity with you, that feel the best in your body, and that are the easiest for you to find. As you learn to work with them, you might notice that your go-to herbs change over time. This is okay! Your herbal preferences will shift and grow along with you.

When it comes to herbal practices for reproductive wellness, my methods and protocols are diverse and customized for each person. Fertility, just like people, can vary from body to body and even over time for the same person. Still, over the years, I've found that there is a specific set of herbs with a strong affinity for the reproductive events that fit under the pregnancy, birth, and postpartum umbrella. These are the herbs I'll introduce you to in *The Herbal Doula*. They include calendula, fennel seed, milky oats, nettle, and more. I'm excited to introduce you to them in ways that will support your reproductive journey. I've benefited tremendously from medicinal herbs during my own experiences with pregnancy endings and fertility challenges, and I've witnessed the special magic of herbs doing their work with countless people.

A note about gender: throughout this book, you will see a pregnant and birthing person referred to with multiple terms. I sometimes use the words *women, pregnant people,* and *folks* interchangeably. I will at times refer to a doula as "she." It doesn't mean that there are no other kinds of pregnant people or doulas, though. Any human with a uterus can be pregnant and give birth, and any human can be a birthworker or doula. Queering language takes time and engaged participation, and I enjoy using a variety of terms, some of which may or may not always resonate with you and your own gender identity.

The Herbal Doula is meant as a guide and helpful reference for all people, but it is not specifically or uniquely focused on the queer, trans, or gender nonbinary experience. Some pregnant and birthing people are indeed women, and many doulas identify as women too. So, throughout this book, you'll see a flow of different pronouns and terms. In the words of clinical herbalist Jessye Finch, "Humans are beautifully complex, and while bodies, sex, and gender have historically been viewed from the perspective of binaries, this kind of framework no longer fits our expansive understanding of the world. To move toward language that feels affirming for all bodies is to directly engage in creating a future that fosters safety, trust, and embodiment."

You will find recipes and food-based remedies in *The Herbal Doula.* All the recipes are highly adaptable. It's common practice to share dietary and nutritional advice when it comes to general wellness tips, and this can be problematic because most popular diet and nutrition advice is based in diet culture, healthism, and fat-phobia. Nutrition advice in holistic circles is also often confusing and based on hype, changes every season, and centers a mishmash of foods that is not rooted in culture or tradition. That's why my books (the guide you hold in your hands as well as my first book, *The Intimate Herbal*) don't offer dietary advice or recommend any dietary restrictions.

As a person of French heritage and with strong cultural traditions in my life and family, I know that my ancestors have leavened grains and cultured milk for centuries, and that my body feels good when I follow their wisdom. I have tremendous respect and love for folks' traditional foodways, and I trust your body's intuition on your cultural foods and everything that's associated with them, like pleasure, memories, and nourishment. As my friend the artist Nicole Gugliotti writes in her zine *Your Body Is Smart,* "Eat food that nourishes you and food that makes you happy. They might be different things sometimes."

I mention food because you'll find recommendations and tips for food-based herbal recipes and preparations in this book. These recipes and tips are meant to be adaptable and accommodating of your favorite ingredients. For example, all milk-based drinks that blend herbs into a yummy beverage could be made from cow's milk, nut milk, oat milk, or any other kind of milk that belongs in your diet. Grains, fats and oils, and vegetables and fruits come in so many variations—go for the ones that are culturally relevant to you and that feel good in your body.

One final thing to note: this guide follows my previous book, *The Intimate Herbal.* If you're looking for a primer on remedy-making herbal practices, body literacy, and cycles, as well as a resource on herbal medicine for beginners, grab a copy of my other book as a companion to *The Herbal Doula.* It's been described as a "treasure trove of herbal goodness" and I know you'll enjoy having it on hand.

In *The Intimate Herbal,* you will dive deep into your capacity for sensuality, libido, fertility, and embodied pleasure through the help of healing herbs and herbal practices. It will be an invaluable addition to your library and, like the thousands of herb-curious folks who now have a copy at home, you'll find answers to all your sexual wellness and medicine-making questions in its pages.

In the years after *The Intimate Herbal* was published, many of my friends and clients entered pregnancy and parenthood. That's when *The Herbal Doula* was born. I look forward to diving into this work with you.

Chapter Overview

Chapter 1. Foundations of Doula Herbalism: Overview of doula herbalism and its practices; the goals and applications of herbs for pregnancy, birth, and postpartum; and a review of modern herb uses.

Chapter 2. Herbal Basics: How to Source Herbs, Store Herbs, and Use Herbs 101. Introduction to types of herbs, types of herbal preparations, and favored herbs for doula herbalism.

Chapter 3. Fertility and Conception: Inclusive strategies for fertility and conception, from intrauterine insemination (IUI) to IVF. Learn how to support fertility with herbal remedies and practices.

Chapter 4. Miscarriage and Abortion: Herbal care for common outcomes of pregnancy. Miscarriage and abortion aftercare include support for uterine spasms or cramping, blood loss, and mood balance.

Chapter 5. Pregnancy and Birth: Simple and safe herbal strategies for common pregnancy ailments like nausea, hemorrhoids, heartburn, vaginal health, and more.

Chapter 6. Postpartum (the Fourth Trimester): How to care for C-section wounds, vaginal tearing, post-birth recovery, mood, and rest with herbs and postpartum practices for nourishment.

Chapter 7. Breastfeeding: Herbs for nipple health and breast health applied as salves and compresses, as well as herbal strategies for milk flow.

Chapter 8. Baby and Child Care: Herbal care for colic, skin rashes, sleeplessness, digestion, and other everyday ailments for babies, toddlers, children, and their parents.

Chapter 9. Herbal Medicine for Doulas and Birthworkers: How to care for yourself as a doula, with herbs and herbal strategies for digestion, stress and anxiety, sleep, and more.

Chapter 10. Doula Herbalism Materia Medica: A selection of safe and accessible herbs used in doula herbalism with the parts used, traditional uses, scientific studies, and home-based recipes for enjoyment.

Chapter 11. Recipes: How to craft delicious herbal remedies for best results, including internal remedies like herbal teas and drinks as well as external remedies for use on the skin.

1

Foundations of Doula Herbalism

What Is a Doula?

A doula is a person who accompanies you during reproductive events. At the core of doula work is a desire to be of service to the health and well-being of the pregnant person and their family. Fertility doulas may support folks along their fertility—or infertility—and conception journeys. Pregnancy doulas support pregnant people from conception to birth. They can assist with physical health and well-being through the relief of prenatal symptoms like nausea or pain, or help with emotional health in addressing anxiety, fear, or low mood.

During birth, the presence of birth doulas is strongly associated with a shorter duration of labor, lower C-section rates (evenly for folks across the income spectrum), and a better overall memory of the birthing experience.[1] A doula can also be present and supportive during miscarriage, stillbirth, or abortion. Some doulas offer full-spectrum care work while others might specialize in one area over another.

Not all doulas are birth doulas, which means that not all doulas offer birth-specific services. So you might find a pregnancy doula to support you during the pregnancy, a birth doula to support the birth, and a postpartum doula to be present in the weeks that follow. You might find one person who does it all, or not. One of the reasons why some doulas may not offer birth support services has to do with accessibility. Being available on call, such as for a birth, isn't suitable for every person, for example if the doula has children of their own at home that need attention and routine, or if the doula has a medical condition or disability that means they need more rest or can't be away from home for long periods.

At its core, a doula is someone who is present to your emotional and physical needs. Doulas can be professionally trained or not. Sisters, aunties, and grandmas have often played the role of doulas to great benefit. A doula is traditionally a nonmedical support person, but some doulas may also have medical training in nursing, midwifery, or in other health care–adjacent fields. Like with any other therapist or wellness provider, it might take a bit of work to find the right doula or doulas for you.

An Introduction to Herbalism and Doula Work

Why invite herbs into conception, pregnancy, birth, and the postpartum period? Herbal medicine and doula work are an awesome match. People have used herbal medicine for pregnancy and birth across time and across cultures. Herbs offer gentle, nourishing, and supportive medicine for the body before, during, and after pregnancy. While it's essential to know herbs well in order to work with them during the reproductive years, avoiding herbs altogether would be unfortunate.

Some safe and simple herbal essentials for conception, pregnancy, birth, and beyond include nourishing nettle infusions for a hearty dose of fertility-promoting vitamins and minerals (including bioavailable iron), ginger as an antiemetic for morning sickness and to prevent vomiting, wound-healing calendula salve for cracked nipples during breastfeeding, and chamomile as a soothing digestive herb for colicky babies. You could do great with only those four herbs. But, of course, you might want to dive deeper into what herbalism has to offer for more targeted actions, which you'll learn in this book.

Building from a solid foundation of simple basic herbal knowhow, herbs can act as supportive therapies for the whole reproductive journey from fertility-building to pre-conception, from conception to pregnancy and birth, and finally from birth and postpartum and caring for both parent and baby. This includes herbal strategies for infertility, miscarriage and abortion, C-section recovery, postpartum depression, and more.

Herbal support doesn't have to be curative—meaning that you implement an herbal protocol as a result of a condition or symptom. Instead, herbal medicine in the context of doula support can be preventive and nurturing. Nourishing infusions can be made to sip on, to soak your feet in, and to enjoy as a compress over the belly or the breasts. Nervous system tonics and mood-lifting herbs can be used as daily, tonifying drinks. Restorative salves and oils can be used to soothe both itchy skin and frazzled nerves or simply to prevent them in the first place. You can take a pleasure-first approach with herbal medicine: taking remedies because they make you feel so good. Pleasure is medicine, and if it's not already a part of your wellness tool kit, you can start including it in your health rituals today.

The safe and informed use of herbal medicine for reproductive wellness doesn't have to be complicated and overly precise to be beneficial. Simple remedies consisting of only a few trusted herbs—from quality sources and prepared with care in the form of food—can do wonders too. As you learn more and develop confidence in your herbal knowledge and abilities, you can find the right approach for your needs. The right approach for you might be a very simple one consisting of only one or two herbs.

Many folks find that they want to start a little garden when their family grows. This can be especially useful if you want to work with medicinal herbs as a way to support your health and the health of your little ones. Herbs like calendula, peppermint, and lemon balm can be easily grown anywhere, even in small pots on the balcony in the summertime. Growing herbs, even if it's just one or two herbs at a time, is a great way to develop your skills as an herbalist and to build relationship with the plant world in a way that will deepen your herbal practice while supporting family health.

Herbalism: Past and Future

The use of herbal medicine, be it from powders, capsules, tinctures and liquid extracts, herbal teas, or other forms, is increasing around the Global North as more people become aware of its benefits. While it may seem like a new phenomenon, the truth is that we are returning to what used to be much more common herbal use of healing plants, seaweed, and fungi. Many of your grandparents or great-grandparents grew up in households where herbal medicine was used in simple daily ways.

It's only in the last hundred years or so that herbal medicine has been erased as a tradition and labeled as inferior medicine. The rise of allopathic medicine, while important and life-saving in many ways, ushered in its wake an era of distrust in herbal medicine, which was soon labeled as unsafe and primitive. It's no coincidence that racism, sexism, and distrust in herbal remedies were successful in making those who use herbal medicine—with a strong tradition of use among women and femmes, those in the Global South and the global majority, as well as with Black, Indigenous, Hispanic, Asian, and other nonwhite folks—seem like their use was rooted in ignorance and folklore. We are now slowly returning to those healing ways as science confirms what earlier herbal practitioners knew to be true.

Still, there are a few threats to herbal knowledge and herbal use today as well as a few lingering biases against herbal remedies. One such threat is the stance that "all herbs are dangerous," which is the other side of the stance that "all herbs are safe," both of which are untrue. Many people who are well educated in medicine but undereducated in herbalism consider plants to be of dubious value. As a result, they may campaign against the use of healing herbs as a whole, and lump all remedies loosely associated with herbal medicine together with other esoteric practices unrelated to herbalism, like homeopathy or astrology. This is especially rampant in medical and scientific circles and leads to patients not disclosing to their doctors the herbs they are taking for fear of being judged.

Numbers are hard to obtain, but it's estimated that more than two-thirds of patients who use herbal remedies as well as supplements won't disclose this to their doctors.[2] Nonwhite folks, low income folks, fat folks, and women are less likely to divulge the herbs they are taking to their doctors because of coexisting and overlapping biases already stacked against them. If people felt more comfortable disclosing the herbs they consume, herb-drug interactions would be more safely handled and fewer people would suffer needlessly.

Another threat to herbalism today is the proliferation of inaccurate and false herbal information—especially from internet sources with low credibility but large reach. This includes information from the "all herbs are safe" camp, which is just as harmful as the belief that all herbs are worthless or dangerous. As an herbal teacher and researcher, I have to parse through *so much* bad information from so many different outlets in order to find reliable and trustworthy herbal profiles that I'm reluctantly inclined to agree with the crowd that doesn't trust herbal medicine because the false information—like the kind found on the internet and social media, for example—can, in fact, be dangerous, especially as it relates to fertility and pregnancy. Unfortunately, the immense amount of false information about herbs online and elsewhere contributes to this fear-mongering.

The solution isn't to stop using herbs, but quite the opposite. Collectively we will all benefit from studying herbs more, from making herbalism accessible, and from separating fact from fiction through education and skill-sharing. Cocreating herbal gardens, sharing remedies, tending to community apothecaries and lending libraries, and gathering together in small groups for seasonal herb walks can all contribute to a better understanding of herbs and how they work through simple, accessible ways.

Ironically, discrediting herbs and herbal medicine contributes to a proliferation of dangerous marketing hype and results in more misuse of herbs, not less. That's because the space that herbalists would occupy in the field of herb care is taken over instead by folks looking to capitalize on people's distrust of conventional medicine while profiting off people's trust in herbs. This is especially relevant in the realm of reproductive health, when folks—like those struggling with infertility or recurrent miscarriage, for example—are in a state of deep vulnerability and looking for support.

Still, so many herbalists today are working on the sidelines collecting information, case studies, and lived experience of herbs as a tool for collective health and liberation. Passionate herbalists are volunteering hundreds and thousands of hours to the study of plants and to the service of their communities through herbal medicine. People who practice traditional herbal medicine passed down from their ancestors have to fight to continue to do so in sustainable ways and to be recognized as valid practitioners. There is tremendous potential for collaborative medicine to emerge in the future, one in which folks who want to work with herbs are invited and welcomed to do so in safe and informed ways.

Plant medicine is a healthy part of our communities. It's a legitimate practice that is both backed by science and by tradition. It exists everywhere around the world and has evolved across cultures and generations. People—and especially women—are drawn to medicinal herbs and want to use them for daily health support and prevention for themselves and their whole families. This is especially true in the realm of pregnancy, birth, postpartum, and baby and child care.

Women have been and continue to be the main users of herbal medicine across genders.[3] Women tend to be the ones who play the role of caretakers for their families and communities. According to Oxfam, women and girls undertake more than three-quarters of unpaid care work in the world.[4] Much of this invisible labor is related to caring for their families' health. Women enjoy working with herbs because herbs are effective for minor health concerns as well as for prevention against mild illnesses, all while promoting good health, which could include anything like digestion support, sleep aids, mood lifting, and more.

The prevalence of herbal medicine use during pregnancy ranges from 7 percent to as high as 55 percent, based on location, ethnicity, and cultural traditions around the globe. Today, about one in five to one in two women uses herbal medicine during pregnancy.[5]

Folks use herbal medicine during pregnancy for conditions like nausea, constipation, urinary tract infections, anxiety, and edema (fluid retention). The most common medicinal herbs used during and after pregnancy are ginger, peppermint, chamomile, red raspberry leaf tea, fenugreek, and fennel. These herbs offer digestive benefits, soothe colic in babies, and enhance milk flow during breastfeeding.

Young families also benefit from herbal knowledge and practices. Young kids can get sick often, but many of their minor childhood illnesses can be safely managed at home with the help of herbal remedies. At a time when there are shortages of kids' over-the-counter medicines as well as a shortage of doctors and nurses, and when hospitals are overwhelmed and under-resourced, basic herbal knowledge can keep your family (and your friends and neighbors and clients) cared for and well.

Folks also derive a sense of pride and usefulness from their knowledge of herbal medicine. Even small parts of the process, such as being familiar with a plant, either through knowing the name or even as a result of cultivating the plant in their own garden, helps provide a basis of trust for the users of herbal medicine and contributes to their desire to work with herbs for health.

Tradition and family history are also important influences on the motivation for using herbal medicine. Long-standing herbal traditions in families and knowledge handed down generation to generation are often precious and trusted as a result of multigenerational safety and benefit. To conclude, there are many ways to engage with herbal medicine through the processes of pregnancy, birth, and postpartum in ways that will benefit you and your family, friends, and community.

Safety of Herbs and Scope of Practice

When it comes to incorporating medicinal herbs into doula care, you need to follow certain rules in order to be safe. Many herbs are not safe during specific windows of reproductive events and should be avoided during that specific window—like during pregnancy, for instance. However, you don't need to avoid herbs altogether. There are simple guidelines and considerations to keep in mind, and you'll learn these in each section of this book.

In this guide, you will find clear chapters based on each reproductive stage, from fertility-building and pre-conception to pregnancy, birth, and beyond. Each stage will have different herbal recommendations based on what is safe and therapeutic at that time. This includes safe herbal strategies during IVF and during pregnancy as well as herbal care for babies and children, for example.

It is hard to find reliable information about what herbs are safe to use during pregnancy and breastfeeding. Modern advice usually tends to recommend avoiding all herbs, just to be on the safe side. I don't fully agree with this advice, because many herbs have been safely used by countless pregnant people across time and across cultures. What's more, many common ailments during pregnancy—such as nausea, heartburn, and hemorrhoids—can be safely relieved with medicinal herbs. Many pregnant folks want to take herbs and want to address minor ailments at home with their chosen remedies. That being said, I agree wholeheartedly with the importance of being careful and mindful of herb use during pregnancy for safety reasons.

I don't recommend that anyone starts taking new herbs during gestation. Instead, you should incorporate medicinal herbs into your diet and lifestyle prior to conceiving. Find out which herbs feel good in your body and which herbal preparations you like best. Once you become pregnant, you'll already have a few herbs at your disposal that you're used to working with. It's important to be cautious by only using safe herbs during pregnancy. There are many safe herbs available to you during gestation. Ginger, peppermint, and slippery elm are all good pregnancy herbs that you can take internally in the form of infusions or in the form of food, which means that you can ingest them. Other herbs—like calendula, plantain, and St. John's wort—make wonderful herbs to use externally in the form of salves or compresses applied over the skin. These are just a few examples of safe pregnancy herbs and herbal practices that need not be avoided.

Herbs available to you during pregnancy are more limited than at other times, just like other food and drink you might swap or restrict, or find that you no longer crave. But the whole reproductive spectrum consists of much more than pregnancy; pre-conception as well as the postpartum period are two examples of reproductive events that can benefit from a variety of herbs and herbal remedies as well.

Pregnant people will continue to seek herbal remedies to accompany their pregnancies and births. Being told to avoid all herbs doesn't actually help anyone. Instead, it encourages a lack of information and common sense around which herbs are safe, which are unsafe, and why. The types of medicinal herbs helpful during gestation are akin to food. Think of them as nourishing foods and spices, and enjoy them with meals, snacks, and yummy beverages to sip on.

Personally, I can't imagine going through conception, pregnancy, birth, and postpartum *without* herbs. My partner and I have been doing an herbal fertility protocol for a couple of years now in preparation for potentially starting a family sometime in our future. Ashwagandha for sperm health, dandelion root for liver cleansing, schisandra berry for balanced cycles—it feels good to include herbal remedies into different life events.

Many of my best friends who became mothers and parents were excited to craft herbal remedies in preparation for their birth and postpartum recoveries. It was part of the magic and the excitement of entering parenthood and family life. I've enjoyed crafting postpartum care packages for my community as well—friends and clients and loved ones near and far. Even people who had never used medicinal herbs before were astonished to find how effective they can be when their doula or midwife recommended them.

Herbs can improve your fertility levels; they can soothe pregnancy nausea; they can balance bleeding after a pregnancy loss or ending; they can speed up healing of your C-section scar or perineal tearing— sometimes making you heal twice as fast, which is so important! Herbs can also relieve symptoms of colic in your baby and increase milk flow for breastfeeding. The list goes on. I believe that everyone, when they find out they're pregnant, should be sent a little herbal care package with the herbs and herbal remedies that will make their pregnancy, birth, and postpartum gentler.

Herbs and herbal remedies can accompany you along the harder parts of pregnancy and birth, like perineal tears, itchy skin, vomiting, and mastitis—there's so much we aren't prepared for and so much we don't know about pregnancy and postpartum when we enter that part of our lives. If you want to be an herbal doula, you are needed and you will absolutely make a difference in people's lives and in your community.

2

Herbal Basics

If you're new to working with herbs, it's important to get familiar with a few herbal basics. How to source herbs, how to store them, and how to use them are a few important things you'll learn in this section. Types of herbs along with different types of herbal preparations follow, as well as herbal doula essentials to get acquainted with before diving deeper into the practice of doula herbalism.

How to Source Herbs

Sourcing medicinal herbs shouldn't be complicated, but quality varies immensely from one source to the next. I'm often dismayed when I walk into stores and see bulk medicinal herbs that look yellowed and totally lifeless. Many herbs and spices do expire quicker than most folks think—usually about a year or two after being processed and packaged, though it depends on how well it's stored and the type of herb and spice in question.

Whole herbs come in various forms. If you're lucky enough to have a garden in which to grow medicinal herbs, you'll have access to the freshest options. If you grow your own herbs, you need to be careful with the way you harvest your herbs in order to harvest them at the right stage of development, which will be different based on what herb you're harvesting and for which purpose. You also want to ensure you're processing your herbs quickly after harvest in order to dry them properly or turn them into other herbal preparations in a way that keeps the herbs potent. Always label your concoctions and keep your materials clean and tidy to avoid contamination.

If you're new to herb gardening and plant identification, make sure to work with an herbalist to help you confirm that the plants you're using are really the ones you think they are! Misidentifying a plant is more common than you think, and even seed packets from reliable sources can sometimes contain seeds other than the ones on the label. One of the most common mistakes that happen during herb growing and processing is forgetting to label your dried herbs post-harvest. A lot of herbs tend to look rather similar to one another once they've been harvested and dried and put away.

If you buy medicinal herbs rather than grow them yourself, you're more likely to buy them in dried form. Dried herbs can be found either as seeds (like fennel seeds and milky oats, the latter of which are unripe seed pods), leaves (like nettle and peppermint), flowers (like calendula and passionflower), roots (like ashwagandha and dandelion root), or as berries (like schisandra berry). Herbs stay vital longer when they're kept whole; this is especially the case with flowers and leaves, such as calendula and peppermint. Once cut or powdered, dried herbs can lose their potency within as fast as six to twelve months.

Whole dried flowers and leaves can stay good for a year or two based on how well they're stored. Seeds, roots, and berries tend to maintain their potency longer—up to three years or so in the right conditions. If your dried herbs look tired, browned, yellowed, and more pale, it might be a sign that they're no longer potent. Aromatic herbs with strong scents will also lose their scent over time. Compost them when they're past their prime. You can't make good herbal remedies out of expired herbs and spices.

Fresh or dried herbs are used to make herbal preparations like infusions, decoctions, tinctures, and external remedies like herbal oils and salves. Herbal preparations are an excellent way to extend the lifespan of healing herbs and to make them more durable and easier to dose. That's because common ingredients in herbal preparations—like alcohol, vegetable glycerin, olive oil, or beeswax—act as preservatives that help keep herbal benefits active for longer periods.

Aside from sourcing whole herbs, either fresh or dried, you might source ready-made herbal preparations from the store, such as herbal tinctures and capsules. There are lots of options at your disposal, and the abundance of options can sometimes be daunting. Bring an herbalist friend to come shopping with you to help you parse the many options, or ask the staff for recommendations.

There are many good and trustworthy herbal companies out there that make quality products out of well-sourced ingredients. There are also quite a few nutritional product companies that make herbal products that aren't that great—mostly from using less potent herbs or from making the remedies less carefully. Be cautious about shopping online and buying from unknown companies. Your local herbalists are great resources in terms of making herbal remedies for you or directing you toward trusted apothecaries you can buy from.

The most common forms of herbal products you can buy for internal use are tinctures (which are either extracted in alcohol or in alcohol-free vegetable glycerin) or capsules. My preferred remedies tend to be tinctures, because you're less likely to take too much. Many people tend to take too many capsules in the spirit of "more is better," which can lead to complications. What's more, many herbal supplements in capsule form are made with concentrated herb extracts, which may increase the risk of side effects or harm when compared with using the whole herb in simpler forms.

External types of herbal remedies you can buy include herbal oils and salves. Pick products that have a short list of ingredients for best results. For some reason, companies like to make really complicated herbal salves with tons of unnecessary ingredients, and I wouldn't recommend them—especially for conditions like healing a C-section scar after a belly birth, or for applying over the nipples during breastfeeding, or for baby and child care. The only ingredients in an herbal salve should be an extraction oil (most commonly olive oil), herbs, and beeswax. One to three herbs in any salve should be enough; any more herbs could lead to unwanted effects or diminished action.

Sourcing-wise, I recommend that you choose herbs from local, organic, and regenerative gardens whenever possible. Support your local farmers and growers; they need your help to keep growing food and healing herbs in sustainable ways. People who grow in regenerative ways take pride in their farms and gardens. It might even be possible to arrange a farm tour and visit the place where herbs are grown and to learn more about the techniques they use.

As you can probably tell by now, which herbs to use and in which form is highly personal and based on many factors, from personal preference and lifestyle habits and more. As you dive deeper into doula herbalism, you will find the right approach for your needs.

How to Store Herbs

Fresh herbs should be processed right away because they wilt and lose their freshness rather fast. Dry them, tincture them, cook with them—find a way to either consume them right away or turn them into an herbal product with a longer shelf life. Fresh herbs can be kept in the fridge until they're used. They can be kept refrigerated anywhere from one day to a week, based on which herb and herb part you're working with. Fresh leaves and flowers should be used quickly, whereas fresh roots and berries might stay fresh longer.

Once dried, medicinal herbs should be kept in a dry spot away from light and moisture. Keep them in sealed plastic bags or glass jars. Make sure to label everything, even though you think you'll remember what they are. On the labels, I write the plant name, the part used, as well as the year. Depending on how large your collection of herbs grows, you might dedicate a pantry shelf to your stash, or a whole pantry. Dried medicinal herbs can last up to a year or two. You can generally tell when they're past their prime because the color will fade and the smell will change over time. As dried herbs age and lose their potency, their smell becomes much less fragrant, to the point of smelling like nothing much. When the herbs are past their prime and no longer good to use, they might have a damp and earthy smell, like an old attic. Toss these in the compost.

Herbal powders have the shortest shelf life and should be consumed within six to twelve months or so for best results. They won't necessarily go bad, but their potency will be much reduced. Tinctures and capsules, on the other hand, tend to stay potent for many years—with tinctures being by far the most stable form of herbal preparation for long-term potency thanks to the preservative powers of alcohol.

Herbal oils can stay good for about a year or two. But because they are oil-based, they will eventually go rancid. Herbal salves, on the other hand, are stabilized by the addition of beeswax—a preservative that lengthens their shelf life—which means they can often last up to two or three years.

Herbs and herbal remedies don't stay fresh forever, and it's essential that you keep an eye on your home apothecary to ensure all of your supplies are fresh and potent. Label all of your personal homemade remedies and date them so you know when they expire. Keep your store-bought remedies in their original containers so you can see their expiry date and ingredient list. Keep your herbal pantry well organized and tidy, and keep your medicine-making material and supplies clean. These simple tips will ensure that your practice of doula herbalism is safe and helpful.

How to Use Herbs

Most folks turn to herbs when they experience a mild symptom or condition that they want to address. Knowing which herb and which herb part to turn to for a specific symptom requires some herbal knowledge. Still, once you've chosen which herb to take, there will continue to be some experimentation in order to find the right herbal preparation for you—an infusion, a tincture, capsules, or other—as well as the right dosage. There are so many ways to use herbs, and the right way to use herbs is the one that works best for you. Start with the simpler formulation and the smallest dosage and go from there.

Aside from using herbs to address a symptom or condition, you might want to explore using herbs as a preventative measure and as a simple lifestyle habit. That's the difference between curative herbal care and preventative herbal care. Curative herbal care seeks to address a condition. Preventative herbal care focuses on gentle tonic herbs like nettle, milky oats, reishi mushroom, and other herbs that can be taken regularly and over the long term for overall wellness. This also includes herbal strategies and practices that are food-based, like using medicinal herbs and spices in food preparation, as well as enjoying herb baths and soaks. These herbal preparations aren't used to address a specific health issue or concern, but rather just for pleasure, enjoyment, and wellness.

How do you choose which herb to use? Aside from herbal knowledge, a few factors can be taken into consideration when it's time to choose which herbs you want to work with. Safety is number one. Choose herbs that have been harvested by a professional to avoid contamination or misidentification. Stick to safe and gentle herbs that have no negative interactions with your current medication. A clinical herbalist can help you assess this. Also, if you're trying new herbs, be sure to pay attention to immediate physical changes that may indicate an allergy. These may include digestive discomfort like cramping, hives or other rashes on the skin, or any changes to your mood or mental energy. For example, I have sensitive skin and so I'm always cautious when I try a new herb as a topical remedy applied to my skin. I'll use a formula that contains a single herb at a time, so that I can assess if I'm having an allergic reaction. If I used a blend of new herbs at once, I wouldn't be able to pinpoint which might cause a reaction in the case of an allergy.

Accessibility and availability are other important factors to consider when choosing which herbs to use. Are the herbs you want to use easy to find and affordable to you? Local herbs or herbs with a history of use in your family, culture, or community can also be particularly well suited to you. Be prepared to experiment and take some time to find the right herbs for your needs. Some herbs are fast-acting, whereas others tend to take longer before their effects are felt.

When folks start working with herbs, they generally find that some herbs and herbal preparations appeal to them more than others. Your preferences may change over time and as you continue working with your herbal protocols. You can adjust dosage and preparation type at any time.

There is one common mistake I see my herbal clients doing when it comes to using medicinal herbs: They take too many herbs at once based on current trends. I can't emphasize enough that social media and online culture pushes new herbs all the time and that it's normal to get caught up in the hype. They all promise to heal us and make us better, *for real this time.* But chasing herbal trends is no long-term solution to feeling unwell, and it will not make us feel better. Building connection and relationship with certain herbs over time, whether or not the herb is trendy, can offer longer-lasting benefits. Trendier herbs can also cost much more than other herbs with similar actions and properties, which makes herbal medicine less accessible to many people in these times of rising cost of living and widespread poverty.

Some folks enjoy buying and consuming trendy herbal remedies. If that's you, and you can comfortably afford it, that's fine! But if you're noticing that the remedies aren't delivering the results you hoped, and if you're routinely consuming many herbs and mushrooms every day while not seeing their benefit, it might be time to simplify your herbal routine and cut back on some of the pricey herbal supplements. There is such a thing as taking too much at once.

This brings us to another important consideration when it comes to how to use herbs: knowing when *not* to use herbs. Medicinal herbs are great additions to your life and health, but they're not a magical solution to every woe. They're living beings that occupy a role in their ecosystems and that exist for multiple purposes outside their medicinal value to humans. Medicinal herbs don't replace access to reproductive services and health care; they don't replace the need for safe and affordable housing and nutritious foods.

Additionally, some health conditions and ailments may warrant medical care rather than herbs. This is especially important in the realm of fertility, miscarriage or abortion, pregnancy and birth, postpartum care, and the health of babies and toddlers. Nurses, midwives, and doctors can help you too. Herbs work best when they're part of a multipronged approach that includes many layers of care, prevention, and treatment.

Types of Herbs

The types of herbs you'll find in the practice of doula herbalism include tonic herbs, nutritive herbs, adaptogen herbs, mood-lifting herbs, and nervine herbs.

Tonic herbs provide energy and general support. They tend not to focus on a single organ or body system but rather to balance the whole body, which makes them good herbs to take regularly and over long periods. Tonic herbs include nettle, milky oats, and reishi mushroom.

Nutritive herbs are rich in bioavailable vitamins and minerals. They're ideal during periods of fatigue or following a big event, like during the postpartum period or after a miscarriage. Nutritive herbs include alfalfa, nettle, and maca.

Adaptogen herbs provide protection against the effects of stress. They increase resilience and support the hypothalamus-pituitary-adrenals (HPA) axis. Some adaptogens have anti-anxiety benefits. Adaptogen herbs include ashwagandha, holy basil, and schisandra.

Mood-lifting herbs help relieve symptoms of anxiety and mild depression. They are useful during conditions like infertility or pregnancy endings. They're nonaddictive and offer relief in gentle ways. Mood-lifting herbs include damiana, holy basil, and lemon balm.

Nervine herbs support the nervous system. They can calm and soothe or energize and uplift. They're helpful herbs for folks under a lot of stress or who experience low energy, fatigue, restlessness, or agitation. Nervine herbs include milky oats, passionflower, and ashwagandha.

Other important herbs in the doula herbalism praxis are herbs used externally for skin and wound healing, such as calendula and plantain, which are both anti-inflammatory herbs with strong benefits for parents and children alike.

Types of Herbal Preparations

The types of herbal preparations you'll find in doula herbalism include infusions and decoctions, compresses, herbal baths and soaks, tinctures, herbal powders, and herbal oils and salves. I don't include herbal capsules here because they're the type of herbal preparation you would likely buy and not make at home.

Infusions are herbal teas made from infusing plants in water. They're typically made with hot water or boiling water and infused for a few minutes, but you can also slowly infuse herbs in cold water as well, most commonly overnight. Herbal infusions are quick and easy to make and are ideal for leaves and flowers as well as some seeds. Infusions will last for one to three days in the fridge. Typical dosage is about one to two cups per day. Medicinal herbs that make good infusions include nettle, peppermint, holy basil, lemon balm, fennel seeds, and milky oats. For roots and berries as well as mushrooms like reishi, you'll want to do a decoction instead.

Decoctions are herbal teas made from simmering plants in hot water or boiling water for up to an hour or a few hours. Decoctions are similar to infusions, except that you use a decoction for any plant material that's harder to extract, like ashwagandha root or reishi mushroom. Decoctions form the basis for delicious healing broths. Decoctions will last up to three to five days in the fridge. Typical dosage is about one to two cups per day. Decoctions can be turned into syrups by mixing them in equal parts with a sweetener like cane sugar or honey, which lengthens its shelf life.

Compresses can be used from either infusions or decoctions. Compresses are simple herbal preparations that consist of dipping a cotton cloth in the herbal tea of your choice and applying the tea-soaked cloth over an area of the body, such as the breasts or the lower belly. It's a good way to administer something similar to an herbal bath or soak in situations where soaking the body or a body part in herbal tea isn't accessible, like if someone is on bed rest or in small restricted spaces with no access to a bathtub.

Herbal baths and soaks are lovely ways to enjoy herbal medicine at home. Herbal infusions or decoctions are poured into the bathtub or into a large vessel to soak in. You can soak the whole body, or just the feet or hands or lower body. Herbal baths and soaks are great remedies for folks who prefer not to consume herbal products through the mouth. This makes herbal baths and soaks ideal for people with digestive issues or chronic nausea, as well as for toddlers and children who enjoy baths.

Tinctures are popular herbal remedies that come in liquid form, typically in 50-mL bottles with a dropper for easy dosing. They're most commonly made in alcohol, which extracts herbal constituents well. You can also craft or find tinctures made with vegetable glycerin, which functions similarly to alcohol (though it extracts some constituents to a lesser degree) while offering a great alternative for folks who don't consume any alcohol, be it for religious, medical, or other reasons. Typical dosages for tinctures are about 1 mL to 3 mL per dose. Tinctures last for many years, thanks to the preservative power of alcohol.

Herbal powders can be used to add to drinks and food. You're probably already familiar with turmeric powder, which you might use in cooking. Other popular powders used in doula herbalism include maca powder, ashwagandha root powder, and shatavari powder. These can be used to make bliss balls, blended with the nut butter of your choice and honey to taste. They get rolled into small balls and are kept in the fridge. Eat one or two bliss balls per day. Herbal powders can also be used to make yummy drinks; add ½ teaspoon herbal powder to the milk of your choice, sweetened to taste. Blend and enjoy. For best results herbal powders should be used within six to twelve months because they lose their potency faster than other types of herbal preparations.

Herbal oils and salves are external remedies meant to be used over the skin. Herbal oils are made by macerating plant material, either fresh or dried, into oil (most commonly olive oil), then left to infuse for two to six weeks in a cool place away from direct sunlight, then strained and bottled. Herbal oils can be used over the skin and as compresses. Herbal salves, on the other hand, are made by blending herbal oils with beeswax. The mixture is heated gently until well combined, then poured into salve jars. The jars are allowed to cool completely before the top lid is sealed. The benefit of adding beeswax to herbal oils and turning them into salve is that it lengthens the shelf life of the infused oil and makes it easier to apply to the skin. Herbal salves are used for minor wounds and to speed skin healing and prevent infections. Salves are valuable during postpartum and for baby and child care.

Herbal Doula Essentials

There are a few medicine-making essentials you'll want on hand in order to craft herbal remedies at home. Below are some of the most important ingredients and tools you'll want at your disposal.

Olive oil is used for infused herbal oils and salves. You don't need a fancy culinary olive oil because the remedies made with it will only be used externally over the skin and not actually ingested. I buy mine in large cans at the grocery store and store them in my herb pantry. Can you use other types of oil? Of course. Olive oil is often recommended because it is shelf-stable and holds itself well once infused with herbs, compared with other types of oil that can go rancid more quickly.

What's more, olive oil tends to be more affordable than other types of oils, such as jojoba or almond oil. It is also well tolerated by a large variety of skin types, even for folks with sensitive skin or various skin allergies. Common herbs infused in olive oil in the practice of doula herbalism include calendula, comfrey, plantain, and St. John's wort.

Beeswax is used for making herbal salves. Once melted into warm infused oils, beeswax then cools and solidifies, turning an oil into a salve that can be more easily applied over the skin. I recommend that you buy beeswax in small chips or discs rather than as a whole block. That's because big blocks of beeswax are hard to cut into, which makes salve-making a bit more strenuous. Small chips or discs of beeswax, on the other hand, are easy to measure and add to a pot of warm infused oil in just the right ratio. Beeswax is a highly stable ingredient and will stay fresh for years. Consider buying beeswax from local small-scale beekeepers in your area.

Alcohol is used for making herbal tinctures. Go for something like vodka or brandy, bought in regular liquor stores. Alcohol is poured over fresh or dried herbs and left to infuse in a tightly sealed jar, away from direct sunlight, for two to six weeks. The resulting tincture is then strained in order to remove the plant material, and stored in glass bottles that have been labeled properly. Because alcohol is such a reliable preservative, well-crafted herbal tinctures will stay fresh and potent at room temperature for years, even decades. Common herbs infused in alcohol in the practice of doula herbalism include milky oats, dandelion root, and damiana.

Vegetable glycerin is another great staple to have on hand for medicine making. It's an alternative to alcohol for making tinctures, but even if you do consume alcohol-based tinctures, you might still want to make *glycerites* as well—that's what we call tinctures made from vegetable glycerin. Vegetable glycerin is a naturally sweet-tasting liquid that's often used for making tinctures for folks who don't consume any alcohol, including those who avoid alcohol for religious or medical reasons, for sober alcoholics who don't want any alcohol in their houses or in their bodies, as well as for children.

Glycerites are also ideal for pregnant folks as well as during breast-feeding. The sweet taste of glycerites makes them ideal for young kids. Vegetable glycerin is poured over fresh or dried herbs and left to infuse in a tightly sealed jar, away from direct sunlight, for two to six weeks. Some people choose to add a small amount of water to the extraction as well. The resulting glycerite is then strained in order to remove the plant material, and stored in glass bottles that have been labeled properly.

Because vegetable glycerin is a good preservative, well-crafted glycerites will stay fresh and potent at room temperature for years. Common herbs infused in vegetable glycerin in the practice of doula herbalism include chamomile and lemon balm.

Other materials to have on hand for an herbal pharmacy include tea strainers, cheesecloth, amber glass bottles, labels, and a few more tidbits described below.

Tea strainers are an essential kitchen tool that any herbal doula will want in their tool kit. Keep a few tea strainers in different shapes and sizes for straining anything from a cup of herbal tea or a cup of herbal tincture to a large pot of infusion for an herbal bath.

Cheesecloth is also a handy tool for straining tinctures or glycerites; place a lining of cheesecloth over a fine mesh sieve and strain your concoctions through.

Amber glass bottles with or without droppers are used for storing and administering tinctures and glycerites. Small glass jars are used for salves. You'll also need lots of glass jars or various sizes for storing all the tinctures and oils that are currently in the process of infusing.

Keep labels on hand; they can be found in most office supply stores.

Folks with gardens might want to invest in herb dryers or dehydrators for drying fresh herbs.

Finally, your herbal doula apothecary will contain many herbs and spices, including some seaweed and mushrooms. Dried flowers to keep on hand include calendula, passionflower, and rose. Leaves include peppermint, nettle, and holy basil. Roots include dandelion, ashwagandha, and shatavari. Powders include maca, turmeric, and chlorella. Seeds include fennel seeds and fenugreek, while berries include schisandra and elderberry. Mushrooms to keep on hand include reishi and shiitake. You'll learn more about each of these herbs and ingredients in the following chapters, along with how to use them for fertility, postpartum, and baby and family care.

Introduction to Doula Herbs

Essential herbs in doula herbalism include ashwagandha, calendula, comfrey, damiana, fennel seed, holy basil, milky oats, passionflower, peppermint, plantain, red raspberry leaf, reishi mushroom, shatavari, and St. John's wort.

Ashwagandha is an adaptogen and general tonic. It's helpful for improving sperm health as well as for lowering anxiety. Ashwagandha is used in doula herbalism for increasing male fertility, for relieving postpartum anxiety, and as an anxiolytic following a pregnancy loss.

Calendula is a medicinal flower used externally over the skin. It is wound-healing, antibacterial, and antifungal. It's used for soothing injection sites during IVF, for mild vaginal infections during pregnancy, and as a topical healing balm for diaper rash in babies.

Comfrey is a wound-healing herb used externally as an oil or salve. Blended with calendula, comfrey is used post-birth and during postpartum healing for perineal recovery from tears, episiotomy, or C-section. It's also helpful in the topical treatment of pregnancy-related hemorrhoids.

Damiana is a mood-lifting nervine herb. It's used for relieving anxiety and depression related to pregnancy endings, be it miscarriage or abortion, as well as during postpartum depression or mild baby blues. Damiana can also support emotional balance during infertility challenges.

Fennel seed is a digestive herb with many benefits for parents and children alike. Taken internally, it soothes colic in babies, increases milk flow during breastfeeding, and relieves tummy aches, gas, and constipation in young children.

Holy basil is a gentle nervine and adaptogen. It relieves stress and anxiety, which makes holy basil useful after miscarriage or abortion, as well as during postpartum recovery. It's also a nice digestive herb, and increases milk flow during breastfeeding.

Milky oats are a restorative nervine herbs. They're used for the stress, anxiety, and mild depression associated with infertility, pregnancy loss, and the postpartum period. Milky oats can also offer benefits to tired parents of young babies and toddlers.

Passionflower is a nervine and soothing herb for the nervous system. It's known to lift mood and give comfort to frazzled hearts and minds. Passionflower is helpful following a miscarriage or during the postpartum baby blues.

Peppermint is a lovely digestive herb. It's refreshing and energizing, and has been used to relieve pregnancy-related nausea. Peppermint can also be used with young children to improve digestion and soothe tummy aches and gas.

Plantain is a healing weed with benefits for skin health and the digestive system. Used externally in the form of compress, soak, oil, or salve, plantain relieves swelling and inflammation. Internally, plantain is helpful with pregnancy-related heartburn as well as with colic.

Red raspberry leaf is a traditional uterine tonic used for relieving spasms and cramping in the uterus. Used externally, red raspberry leaf acts as a toner and astringent, which makes it ideal for external application to relieve pregnancy-related hemorrhoids and varicose veins.

Reishi mushroom is an adaptogen and tonic. It supports immunity and liver health. Traditionally taken as a tea, reishi is a general tonic during infertility, following pregnancy endings, and during the postpartum period.

Shatavari is an adaptogen with an affinity for the female reproductive system. It has been shown to assist with fertility as well as supporting mood balance during postpartum. Shatavari is a galactagogue, which means it increases milk flow during breastfeeding.

St. John's wort is used for wounds and skin healing. It has been shown to speed healing of C-section scars and can aid in the repair of perineal tearing during postpartum recovery.

3

Fertility and Conception

Fertility-building and pre-conception strategies with herbs are beneficial in many ways. I recommend fertility-building to most folks, regardless of whether they are facing infertility or low fertility. Fertility-building means supporting the health of the reproductive system. More than that, fertility-building also means paying attention to the hormonal system, the nervous system, to digestion and immune health and body literacy. In other words, it means tuning in to your body and mind and heart in nourishing, restorative ways.

Fertility is the ability to conceive by combining an egg with sperm. A person or couple is believed to be fertile when they conceive without assistance within twelve months of inserting sperm into the vagina (either through sex or other means) during the ovulation period. Some people get pregnant right away! Fertility challenges occur when conception does not happen after a period of more than twelve months.

Queer couples and single parents may have a different approach to conception. For example, they might start directly with uterine insemination (IUI), either in a clinic or at home. But our relationship to fertility remains the same no matter how conception happens and through which means. No matter how you conceive, it can sometimes take longer than you expected. Many people have conceived after eighteen months, two years, four years . . . And some people don't conceive without assistance.

You can commit to a fertility-building herbal protocol prior to trying to conceive. And if you've been trying to conceive for more than six months and your efforts haven't resulted in a pregnancy, you might want to take a break from attempting to conceive and focus on fertility-building instead.

Taking a break from trying to conceive can seem counterintuitive when you're so focused on your baby-making goals. But it's really important to reassess your needs and your timeline when you feel your mental health becoming affected by your fertility challenges. Trying to conceive can take a heavy toll on your emotions, especially when the process lasts longer than you'd imagined.

Even though fertility challenges can seem like a setback, they can actually expand your capabilities, both in therapeutic settings and in your personal life. People experiencing infertility might prefer to work with a doula who has experienced what they are going through. As much as folks idealize and idolize wellness as the absence of discomfort, the truth is that setbacks make you more empathetic, more compassionate, and oftentimes, wiser.

If you've experienced or are experiencing difficulties along your conception journey, it could be your gift as a doula (and friend, and accomplice, and ally), rather than your personal failure, as some of us tend to view our journeys to parenthood when they're long and difficult. Conception is a morally neutral physiological event, and difficulty conceiving doesn't mean there's anything wrong with you.

Trying to Conceive and Fertility-Building

If you're first trying to conceive, whether that's through sex or via IUI, you'll want to chart your menstrual cycle and identify when you're ovulating. Track your basal body temperature, your cervical position and mucus, and other ovulation symptoms so you can identify a pattern and guess when ovulation is about to happen. You can also use ovulation strips. Plan sex in the days leading up to ovulation and on ovulation day.

Your menstrual cycle follows the same four phases every time: menstruation, follicular phase, ovulation, and luteal phase. The ovulation phase only lasts twenty-four hours, so you want to time it well. You're considered to be fertile for several days in each menstrual cycle because, even though the ovulation phase lasts only one day, sperm can remain active for several days before ovulation. So a good time to insert sperm into the vagina would be in the few days before ovulation.

Tending to your fertility in a holistic way means taking care of yourself. Stress can negatively affect fertility, as can lack of sleep and low-nutrient diets (including not eating enough calories). If your menstrual cycle has been all over the place and irregular, or too short, fertility-building means getting involved in balancing your hormones and cycle. Boosting egg quality and sperm quality is also important during fertility-building.

Herbs for egg and sperm development and quality include maca, nettle, shatavari, and ashwagandha. Maca is an adaptogen and increases libido and fertility for folks of all genders. Nettle is a nutritive tonic and is specifically useful for women's fertility. Shatavari is an adaptogen and increases vaginal lubrication while supporting egg quality. Ashwagandha is an adaptogen and improves sperm health. Take these regularly for at least three months.

Aside from supporting the reproductive system, fertility also benefits from supporting the body as a whole. So you might increase your intake of nutritive tonic herbs like oat straw and alfalfa. You can add gentle liver tonics to your daily regimen as well: schisandra berry and reishi mushroom come to mind. Herbs to heal and nourish the nervous system often support fertility, too. Milky oats are phenomenal allies for the nervous system, and other calming and mood-lifting herbs include passionflower, lemon balm, and damiana.

Use this protocol (nutritive herbs, nervines, and mood-lifting herbs) during the pre-conception period in order to support healthy fertility. People of all genders can benefit from this herbal support. Consider a minimum of three months and up to a year of fertility-building herbal support prior to conception for best results. Pre-conception care has been associated with better pregnancy and maternal health outcomes.[1] Taking the time to tune in to your body and provide your body with increased nourishment in the period before conception can do wonders for your health and fertility.

I like to think of tending to fertility as being like tending to a garden. With daily care and nourishment, you have the potential to help create an environment in which life thrives. Like in a garden, once the soil is balanced and full of nutrients and healthy microorganisms, sometimes all you have to do is throw in a handful of seeds and watch them bloom.

What Affects Fertility

Folks have noticed that some lifestyle changes may sometimes lead to better fertility. You might want to experiment with these and see what it does for you, though these recommendations should also be taken with a grain of salt. Common advice suggests having children younger (under age thirty-five), reducing tobacco and alcohol use, keeping a balanced exercise routine (excessive exercise may be linked to lower fertility), and maintaining a healthy weight (not too underweight and not too overweight).

There have been quite a few wide-reaching discussions about weight and what is considered a healthy weight. The main argument centers on who decides what a healthy weight is. Using body mass index (BMI) as a standard has been deemed racist for many reasons, as determined by the American Medical Association. I personally don't use BMI as a health measure in my practice. What is a healthy weight? I suggest consulting your health care provider to determine a healthy weight for your body type.

As a practitioner, I'm cautious around this type of lifestyle advice in general but especially when it comes to fertility. I've seen couples who had the most "perfect" diets and lifestyles, and who still struggled with infertility. I've also seen smokers with junk-food diets conceive children effortlessly and go on to experience easy full-term pregnancies and raise healthy children. And as for age, thanks to developments in assisted reproductive technologies, women in their late forties and even their fifties can become pregnant and give birth. As you'll read below, there are many other factors that impact fertility. A health care approach that focuses on individual choices ignores the context we exist within and which includes environmental, relational, and intersectional factors.

Conventional advice around fertility places most of the responsibility on the individual. For instance, many health professionals believe that infertility is caused by advanced age, smoking, drinking alcohol, being overweight or underweight, and either exercising too much or not enough. But blaming individuals for widespread health issues and conditions like infertility is misguided and rooted in ableism. It also disregards the impacts of environmental pollutants on reproductive health, the effects of which have been widely proven by science.

Environmental Pollutants and Fertility

Metals and chemicals in the air, water, food, and common health and beauty products can be damaging to fertility. These accumulative toxins decrease sperm count and function. They are also linked with anovulation and impaired implantation, all of which contribute to infertility. Researchers have noted that this damage may not only decrease natural fertility but also decrease the chances of successful IVF.

The worst contaminants for fertility are endocrine-disrupting chemicals (also known as EDC). They include chlorinated pesticides, polychlorinated biphenyls (PCBs), dioxins, bisphenol A (BPA), and organophosphate pesticides and herbicides such as Roundup. Many of these are known as persistent organic pollutants (POPs). POPs are either currently used or were formerly used in industrial processes and remain in the environment much longer than other chemicals.

Many other chemicals, metals, and air pollutants can lower fertility as well. The list is too long and too boring to mention here, but you can look it up online if you want to learn more. A 2018 meta-analysis published in the *Reproductive Biology and Endocrinology* journal also showed a close association between female infertility and air pollution.[2] Folks living in lower-income neighborhoods tend to be exposed to higher levels of air pollution than those who live in wealthier areas, making poverty a fertility issue. The real takeaway? It's that infertility (and this includes low fertility) is a widespread issue that shouldn't be blamed on individual choices and lifestyles but rather on systemic systems and failures that require collective organizing and radical change.

If you're feeling hopeless or discouraged about the presence of chemicals in our air, food, water, and consumer products—it's normal to be upset! Collective resistance against polluters is the only way forward for a healthier future. The real, long-term solution is to hold companies accountable for their share of pollution through policies, carbon pricing, and just transition. That being said, in the meantime, there are things you can do to protect your fertility with herbs now.

I need to mention again that herbs alone won't heal us, and herbal medicine needs to be paired with collective action against widespread pollution. Still, herbs are pretty amazing, and many herbs have the potential to fight and even reverse some of the damage caused by the pollutants you've been exposed to. Some of the most therapeutic herbs for supporting fertility and reversing the damages of environmental pollutants are also tonic herbs you might already be taking, like turmeric and reishi mushroom.

Let's start with BPA. It's one of the most investigated endocrine disrupting chemicals out there. It's used in plastic bags and plastic packaging, and you've likely been exposed to it throughout your life. BPA exposure is associated with female infertility.[3] It's also linked with PCOS, a common disorder that affects fertility and reproductive health.[4] Moreover, higher levels in BPA are also associated with an increased risk of miscarriage once you do become pregnant.[5] BPA exposure lowers sperm count, and it's been associated with low libido and erectile dysfunction. It all sounds pretty bad, I know, but medicinal herbs can help.

Liver herbs like turmeric and milk thistle can help reduce the risks of BPA exposure. Curcumin from turmeric has been shown to reduce

BPA-induced oxidative stress.[6] Take curcumin in the form of turmeric powder added to food. Turmeric powder is delicious blended with warm milk and honey as a daily drink. Milk thistle seed contains the compound silymarin, which helps lessen the impacts of BPA exposure on the body. You can take milk thistle seed in the form of tincture.

Some adaptogenic herbs can also protect against BPA-induced health concerns. Both astragalus and ashwagandha root, as adaptogens, help protect against the risks of BPA exposure.[7] Their therapeutic impact acts on the brain as well as the liver. Astragalus and ashwagandha can be taken in tincture form for easy dosing, or as powders.

Dioxin exposure is another concern for fertility. Dioxins are a type of widespread POPs found in water, food, and air. Dioxins remain in the body for many years. Both animal studies and human epidemiological studies have shown that exposure to dioxins is linked with long-lasting adverse effects on the male reproductive system, impacting both hormones and semen quality.

You can turn to antioxidant herbs to prevent or reverse the effects of dioxin exposure. Think of herbs like the antioxidant powerhouse turmeric. Curcumin, one of the active compounds in turmeric, helps detoxify the dioxin burden from the body.[8] Enjoy turmeric as an ingredient in food and as a powder mixed with warm milk and honey. Healing mushrooms like reishi also support the body against the risks associated with dioxins. Enjoy reishi in the form of tincture. Dried slices of reishi mushroom can also be used in herbal broths or tea, which is a time-tested way of ingesting it.

Heavy metals and phthalates are other common pollutants associated with lower fertility.[9] For heavy metal chelation, take the microalga chlorella as well as cleansing herbs like milk thistle seed. And finally, to detoxify from phthalates, go for deep liver tonics like milk thistle seed and dandelion root. Take chlorella in the form of tablets. Milk thistle seed and dandelion root can be taken as tinctures.

There are wider commitments we can make as a society that will support fertility and reduce our toxic load. This includes phasing out harmful chemicals from agriculture and industrial processes for a greener future and healthy babies and families for generations to come. The real solution to environmental pollutants isn't a personal commitment to living a "toxin-free" life, which is impossible as a human being on earth, but rather coming together for collective action to hold polluters accountable and reverse the damage that has been done.

After all, as much as we can focus on the effects of pollution on humans and our fertility levels and overall health, the fact is that the same pollutants are also negatively affecting birds, bees, and other pollinators as well as fungi, microbes, bacteria, native plants, seaweed, and every other life form on the planet, all of which we rely on for our own survival.

On a smaller scale, you can support local regenerative farmers and artisans who grow food and craft products in earth-loving ways, if that's available to you. Caring for your body and tending to the land go hand in hand. After all, we're a part of the earth and the earth is a part of us. Fertile bodies and fertile land ask the same thing of us: reciprocal care, nourishment, and safe space in which to grow new life.

Infertility and Difficulty Getting Pregnant

Infertility—the inability to conceive—affects many people today. Up to one in four or five couples experiences infertility. It is not considered to be a disease, but it can be disabling. Infertility can cause complex trauma, and it affects psychological and emotional health. A third of infertility cases are known to be caused by male factors, a third are caused by female factors, and a third are caused by unknown factors. Male or female infertility can be due to physical causes.

Common physical causes of infertility include PCOS, thyroid disorders, and premature ovarian insufficiency (this is when ovarian function declines significantly before the age of forty). Other physical causes include fibroids, blocked fallopian tubes, endometriosis, and low sperm count. Physical or functional issues that affect fertility can be identified in simple lab tests and physical exams.

Identifying a physiological reason for infertility is actually good news. It sounds odd, but it's true! That's because you can address the root cause of infertility and, in many cases, reverse infertility and go on to conceive a healthy child. People might experience either primary infertility or secondary infertility. Primary infertility is when a full-term pregnancy has never been achieved. Secondary infertility is when at least one prior full-term pregnancy has been achieved. Infertility might mean not conceiving, or it might mean not carrying a pregnancy to term (such as miscarrying).

When no factors can be identified for infertility, you have what is frustratingly known as "unexplained infertility." It's a pretty common diagnosis and affects about one in three of all infertility cases. Unexplained infertility is such a bummer. When you deal with infertility with a known cause (blocked tubes, uterine scarring, PCOS, endometriosis, and low sperm count are all common examples), you can take steps to address it. But unexplained infertility takes away your sense of control. Many people find that to be very difficult emotionally. A full third of infertility cases are due to unexplained factors, so it affects a large number of folks.

While there are no herbal protocols absolutely guaranteed to fix infertility, especially when it's unexplained by physiological causes, herbs do help. If you have found a functional reason for infertility, go ahead and follow an herbal protocol specifically geared for that issue.

For example, low sperm count can be improved with ashwagandha and eleuthero. Ashwagandha root benefits testicular health and increases fertility via both stress reduction, higher sperm quality, and higher sperm count. Eleuthero root has been found to increase sperm count and may help relieve impotence or erectile dysfunction while also supporting the health of the body as a whole.

PCOS-related infertility can also be addressed with herbal medicine. Folks with PCOS are at a higher risk of infertility, because PCOS commonly affects ovulation. Many people with PCOS experience anovulation, which means that they don't ovulate regularly. That being said, medicinal herbs can make a difference in increasing fertility and supporting healthy conception and pregnancy for folks with PCOS. Let's talk about the herb vitex, for instance, which is also known as chasteberry.

Vitex is one of the best herbs to improve fertility with PCOS. Vitex is beneficial because it lowers prolactin levels. Prolactin is typically elevated in folks with PCOS and is a leading cause of amenorrhea (lack of menstruation) and infertility. Elevated prolactin can suppress follicle maturation, ovulation, and contribute to ovarian cysts. This makes vitex an excellent herbal remedy in the context of PCOS. Vitex also regulates the menstrual cycle and helps reverse infertility in women with PCOS.

A study showed that vitex supplementation helped lengthen a short luteal phase in women with PCOS.[10] The luteal phase is the part of the menstrual cycle between ovulation and menstruation. Ideal luteal phase length for achieving pregnancy is anywhere from ten to seventeen days. The luteal phase is considered too short if it lasts less than ten days. A short luteal phase can be associated with infertility.

In this study, women with PCOS had a luteal phase of only 3.4 days. In three months of daily treatment with vitex, their luteal phase length grew to a staggering 10.5 days! The dosage was 20 mg per day. Note that vitex isn't for everyone, so work with an herbalist in devising a preconception plan. Other helpful herbs in supporting fertility for folks with PCOS are milk thistle seed, ashwagandha root, maitake mushroom, and schisandra berry.[11]

Another example of herbal treatment for root causes of infertility is with premature ovarian insufficiency (POI), which has also been known in the past as premature ovarian "failure." Words matter—the condition isn't a failure but just an insufficiency, and it can be remedied. Five to ten percent of women with POI are able to conceive without assistance. Chinese herbs were shown to increase pregnancy rates in women with POI. In one such study, ninety women with POI-related infertility followed a three-month-long treatment with Chinese herbs. The herbs included dong quai and codonopsis, among many others. After the treatment, 20 percent of these women conceived and experienced a healthy pregnancy and birth.[11]

There are many examples of using herbs to improve fertility. More generally speaking, fertility herbs like maca and shatavari can increase the chances of conception as well. Maca is an adaptogen and potent nutritive. It is rich in vitamins and minerals. Maca helps increase sperm production, sperm quality, and overall fertility. As a hormone balancer, maca often offers a heightened libido and sexual desire. Shatavari is an adaptogen, aphrodisiac, reproductive tonic, and fertility builder. It helps balance hormones, with an action on the menstrual cycle and pelvic inflammatory diseases. It is known to increase vaginal lubrication. Vaginal lubrication in the form of cervical mucus can support fertility because it encourages the movement of sperm inside the vaginal canal, and offers nourishment to the sperm while it's on its way to the egg. Both maca and shatavari can be taken in the form of powders added to foods, like smoothies and bliss balls.

When it comes to unexplained infertility, there is no one-size-fits-all herbal approach. That being said, I've found in my life and practice that unexplained infertility is really hard on the emotional body and hard on people's moods and satisfaction with life. Unexplained infertility means you have to release expectations and you have to release control. Some herbs have a strong affinity with supporting mental health and emotional health. This includes milky oats, passionflower, lemon balm, and damiana. Milky oats are a potent nervine tonic. Passionflower has an affinity with the emotional heart and is calming. Lemon balm is a stress reliever and digestive herb. Damiana is an euphoriant herb with antidepressant properties. Because pregnancy is possible when dealing with unexplained infertility, these herbs can also be enjoyed in small doses until you have a positive pregnancy test.

Finally, entheogenic plant medicine might be worth investigating for people who are deep in the unexplained infertility hellhole. It's hard to stay positive when something as biologically human as wanting to have a child doesn't work out, month after month, sometimes for years. Women struggling with infertility are more likely to suffer from depression, anxiety, hopelessness, and feelings of worthlessness in life. Infertility has also been linked with suicidal thoughts. If infertility is bringing you symptoms of emotional unease to the point that daily life is becoming hard to manage and enjoy, you might need a break from trying to conceive. Reach out for help and take care of yourself.

It sounds counterintuitive because, if you're trying to conceive, you feel like you have to keep trying every cycle to have every chance on your side that it will result in a healthy pregnancy. But stress may impede fertility. If you're stressed out and depressed, you might actually be lowering your chances of getting pregnant.

Caring for your mental and emotional health is essential. People who've struggled with infertility find that the depressive, anxious thoughts don't just magically go away when you do get pregnant. If you live in a state of anguish and fear during the conception period—especially if that's an extended period of time, sometimes years—you are at higher risk of experiencing a lot of anxiety during your pregnancy as well. It's hard to change psychoemotional patterns, and pregnancy, birth, and the postpartum period all carry the potential to be stressful and trying. You can do what you can to offer yourself the gift of grace. You're not alone in this, even though it might feel that way.

Counseling, community care, and support groups or sharing circles can all do wonders for supporting emotional health during infertility. Along with supportive therapies, I would explore entheogens like mood-altering and psychoactive plants, fungi, and substances. Psilocybin mushrooms, MDMA, LSD, and other types of medicines can open new doors for hope and happiness. The only caveat with those substances is that you have to make sure you're not pregnant when you take them! That means taking a few months off TTC while you plan a session with entheogenic medicines, if that's something that appeals to you and is available.

Sessions with entheogenic medicine can reframe and repattern thoughts and attitudes around infertility. If that's something you'd like to pursue, find a practitioner who's well resourced in that arena. Ceremonies, rituals, and integration are important parts of the healing process. These medicines blend really well with plant medicine like milky oats and damiana too.

The interesting part about working with plant medicine to help lessen the psychoemotional impacts of infertility is that the goal of treatment is to learn to be okay with the experience of infertility. It can increase your capacity to handle hard emotions and circumstances. But here's the thing: lowering stress has been shown to positively impact fertility and improve chances of pregnancy. Whatever the outcome, you can ally yourself with medicinal herbs throughout the journey.

Inclusive Conception

Holistic conception is the act of conceiving a baby through the means that work for you and your body and circumstances. What can conception look like for different folks?

It's generally assumed that conception will take place when two people—one of whom has sperm, and one of whom has eggs—get naked and make love. And indeed conception does happen like that a lot of the time, which is sweet because it is easy, low-cost, and relatively pain-free (depending on your level of pelvic comfort and your reproductive anatomy) compared with other assisted methods of conception. But there are many other ways for conception to happen. Queer people, for example, have used assisted methods of conception for a long time, along with folks who may have experienced medical conditions that make standard conception methods (a.k.a. "natural conception") inaccessible.

The truth is that even healthy able-bodied heterosexual couples also need to use assisted methods of conception sometimes. As infertility cases continue to rise, this will only become more common (and hopefully destigmatized). "Natural conception" is often seen as the ideal way to conceive—meaning with no assistance. But that belief is rooted in ableism and religious dogma, and has the potential to be harmful to health, especially for those people for whom this type of conception is not possible. We need new language to describe unassisted conception and assisted conception, as well as unassisted birth and assisted birth, that go beyond the natural-unnatural binary. There's no such thing as unnatural conception and unnatural pregnancies and births.

Believing in "natural conception" as the main or most valid form of conception ignores the existence of nonheterosexual conception processes, and also dismisses the many folks who carry or care for children,

including lesbian and gay couples, trans people, and gender noncon-
forming people, as well as single folks, women who can't conceive or
carry, those who conceive with donor eggs, people who have had miscarriages, adoptive parents, stepparents, and surrogates. There are a lot
of different ways to experience pregnancy and parenthood.

Honoring people's experiences paves the way for healthy, resilient
families and communities where everyone is welcome. It's important
to note that conceiving via assisted conception usually involves a huge
emotional, physical, and financial investment. Care and support can
make a huge difference in the process.

Assisted Ovulation

This process is called ovulation induction. When you consult for fertility assistance, it's often the first treatment offered once you've com-
pleted your tests and blood work. The process is simple and consists
of five days of medication starting at the beginning of the menstrual
cycle. Ovulation induction will increase the number of eggs released
in that cycle—as the name suggests. If you don't ovulate, it will help
increase ovulation rates, and if you already ovulate, you'll release more.
The logic is that the more eggs you release, the higher your chances of
conception.

Ovulation induction is the most affordable and noninvasive procedure for fertility assistance (aside from medicinal herbs, of course!).
The only drawbacks are that some folks are sensitive to the medication
and can notice unpleasant side effects like mood swings and headaches.
Weight gain is another possible side effect, but weight gain is a neutral
event and is only considered negative because we exist in a fat-phobic
world.

For best results, I recommend a pre-conception herbal protocol last-
ing a minimum of one month and up to three months prior to beginning
ovulation induction. You can follow the protocol outlined in the section
above for egg and sperm quality. Your go-to herbs are ashwagandha,

maca, shatavari, and nettle. If stress is an issue in your life, go ahead and add milky oats, either in the form of herbal infusions or tincture.

Egg Retrieval and Sperm Deposit

Assisted methods of conception include egg retrieval and sperm deposit. This can be done in order to freeze your eggs or sperm as a preventative measure. For example, some of my girlfriends in their thirties haven't met their partners yet but know they want to be mothers. They froze some eggs as an insurance policy because we don't all meet "the one" at the right time. Others have frozen their eggs and later became solo poly moms. There are so many options of what parenthood and family can look like, and egg freezing is a great addition to fertility care.

There are also medical reasons to freeze your eggs. This includes before chemotherapy or radiation therapy in cancer patients, for example. Maybe you have a health condition like endometriosis, PCOS, or uterine fibroids that could impact your fertility. If your family history includes high-risk cancer genes, early menopause, or infertility issues, you might want to freeze your eggs. Or perhaps you've had a series of abnormal Pap tests, or a sexually transmitted infection like chlamydia or gonorrhea, which could impact your ability to get pregnant in the future.

A trans man might also freeze his eggs before undergoing gender transition. The same goes for freezing your sperm. You might freeze your sperm before undergoing chemotherapy or radiation, or before transition. Other common reasons for egg retrieval and sperm deposit include in preparation for reproductive assistance like IVF, where both egg retrieval and sperm deposit will take place.

In terms of herbal support for egg retrieval or sperm deposit, a lot can be done ahead of time to ensure your eggs or sperm are the highest quality they can be. Herbs for egg health include nettle, shatavari, and maca. Herbs for sperm health include ashwagandha and maca. For best results, take these herbs daily for one to three months.

Nettle leaf can be taken as an herbal infusion—drink 1 cup daily. Shatavari (usually for women) and ashwagandha root (usually for men) can be taken in tincture form: take 1–3 mL daily, diluted in juice or water. Maca root is used with folks of all genders and can be taken as a powder added to smoothies and drinks. Go for about 1 teaspoon daily.

Intrauterine Insemination (IUI)

The next step in alternative conception would be IUI. The insemination involves injecting the collected sperm sample into the uterus using a speculum. The injection process can be painless or not. It might cause some discomfort since the speculum is inserted through the vagina and passed to the uterus all through to the cervix, usually without lube. The process itself takes about five to ten minutes, but involves a few visits to the clinic over the days beforehand.

Though IUI doesn't involve egg retrieval, it does include some lab tests, like blood work, and physical tests, like sperm testing and a pelvic exam, to ensure the reproductive system is functioning well.

In preparation for IUI, a sperm sample will be required, from which a semen analysis is done. You can increase sperm quality ahead of the IUI process with daily ashwagandha for about ninety days, or the length of a full sperm cycle (also known as spermatogenesis). Take ashwagandha in the form of capsules or tincture. Aim for a total of 600 mg per day split between two doses, like one with breakfast and one with dinner.

There are interesting herbal strategies to play with when it comes to preparing for IUI. First of all, IUI often involves the use of oral or injectable ovulatory stimulants. You can request an unmedicated IUI cycle, but most fertility clinics prefer to do a medicated cycle with ovulatory stimulants because they can have a higher chance of success.

During IUI, the process of going to the clinic itself can be stressful, and the use of ovulatory stimulant medication can be difficult emotionally if you experience side effects. It can make you weepy, irritable, depressed, or anxious. The typical dosing only lasts a few days, and the side effects dissipate over time, so it's not a long-term problem.

Herbal strategies for unmedicated IUI are centered around regulating the menstrual cycle and preparing the body for ovulation. Herbs like maca and shatavari act as reproductive tonics and offer adaptogenic properties as well. Maca and shatavari powder can be mixed into bliss balls with nut butter. Eat one or two balls per day, or about the equivalent of 1 teaspoon of powdered herbs per day. Nervine herbs like milky oats will help nourish the nervous system, and mood-lifting herbs like damiana can assist with low mood and symptoms of irritability or anxiety. Milky oats extract well as an herbal tea—you can blend them with nettle tea and peppermint for a yummy sip. Take damiana as a tincture, a few drops as needed.

During a medicated IUI, you need to keep herbs to small, intentional doses. Small cups of nettle and milky oats tea can be sipped on, along with peppermint and ginger. I recommend avoiding any herbs that are new to you at this time as well as any herb that isn't pregnancy-friendly, since you could be pregnant any day now.

In Vitro Fertilization (IVF)

Many folks conceive through IVF. It is not a single procedure but a multiple-step process. First, you increase egg production with injectable ovulatory stimulants. Next, you have an egg retrieval via follicular aspiration and a sperm deposit. The mature eggs are fertilized with the sperm in a lab. Following more hormone treatment, the healthy embryo or embryos are then implanted into the uterus in what is called an embryo transfer. A full IVF cycle takes about two months. If the first cycle was unsuccessful, you can repeat the embryo transfer. You'll probably want to prepare mentally, emotionally, and physically for IVF, and herbal medicine is a great way to nourish your body in preparation for it.

Herbs for IVF include nutritive herbs like nettle and oat straw. These are best enjoyed as daily infusions. Nervine herbs that support the nervous system include milky oats and lemon balm. Medicinal mushrooms like reishi act as general tonics and can be enjoyed in the form of an infusion.

Like IUI, IVF can be done unmedicated, which means without fertility drugs. But it's really rare to go that route because the success rates are lower than with stimulated IVF. Because the cost of IVF can be prohibitive for most folks, they'll often choose to go the medicated route because they find it may increase their chances of conceiving during that cycle.

The main conditions that folks currently undergoing IVF will need support with are mood-balancing and anxiety, digestive support, and overall comforting. Injectable hormones involved in the IVF process can make you moody. Aside from mood swings, the fertility medications can also cause cramping, bloating, digestive upset, and nausea along with weight gain, commonly up to ten pounds. The injection site may get irritated, with localized redness, itching, or swelling.

Herbs for IVF include soothing digestive herbs like fennel, chamomile, and ginger. They can help lessen symptoms of bloating, nausea, and stomach cramps. You might want to keep topical remedies on hand too: calendula salve or other herbal salves like plantain can be applied over the injection site to soothe irritation and itch.

You want to keep herbal strategies simple and safe during an IVF cycle. Take herbs in the form of infusions (a.k.a. herbal teas) rather than tinctures or capsules. Possible infusions include nettle, milky oats, fennel, chamomile, and ginger. Compresses are great. You can soak a facecloth in chamomile tea and apply the warm tea-soaked cloth over your face or forehead for a moment of relaxation. You might have achieved a pregnancy, so stick to pregnancy-friendly herbs and remedies from this point on.

In the event of an unsuccessful IVF cycle, after which you haven't become pregnant, many herbal strategies would be helpful for your body and mind. Enjoy calming and restorative adaptogen herbs like ashwagandha; liver tonics like milk thistle seed, schisandra, and turmeric; and gentle mood-lifters like passionflower and blue vervain. A journey with infertility doesn't always end with a pregnancy. There are many other ways to become a parent, including surrogacy and adoption.

Considerations for Using Herbs During Assisted Fertility

Before and during assisted fertility and conception, you'll want to be mindful of the herbs you work with. Avoid herbs that could be negatively affecting your menstrual cycle, ovulation process, or sperm-making. If you're unsure, consult with a clinical herbalist and follow their recommendations. Be careful with herbs that affect hormones. It's important to start with fertility-building protocols for a minimum of one month and ideally three months prior to assisted conception processes. Fertility-building herbal protocols include herbs in the form of tinctures, herbal teas, and soaks.

Once it's time for egg retrieval, sperm deposit, ovulation induction, or IUI, you'll want to go easy on the herbs and let the process unfold with minimal herbal intervention. You can consume small amounts of herbal tea made from safe herbs. I don't recommend that you introduce new herbs to your routine during assisted fertility treatments. That's why it's so helpful to start working with herbs earlier in the fertility process—months or years before you enter fertility work.

In preparation for IVF, you can follow fertility-boosting protocols for a minimum of one month and ideally three months or more prior to beginning an IVF cycle. Stop herbal treatment one month prior to starting your IVF cycle, unless you're under the care of a clinical herbalist who's working in collaboration with your fertility care team. In the event of a successful IVF cycle, safe and gentle pregnancy herbs are now available to you. And in the event of an unsuccessful IVF cycle, the medicinal herbs listed in the following pages have a lot to offer you and are safe to consume.

Medicinal Herbs for Fertility and Conception

Ashwagandha is a traditional remedy of Ayurveda. It's an adaptogen and pro-fertility herb. It improves fertility by supporting healthy eggs and sperm production. Ashwagandha is one of the best herbs you can take for sperm quality. Because the full sperm regeneration cycle (spermatogenesis) is about two to three months, you'll want to make sure to do a full ashwagandha protocol that is at least that long. In a study on the fertility effect of ashwagandha in infertile men, there was a 167 percent increase in sperm count, 53 percent increase in semen volume, and 57 percent increase in sperm motility after ninety days of treatment with ashwagandha.[12]

It's also an adaptogen herb, which means it lessens the impacts of stress on the body. This includes the impacts of emotional, mental, and environmental stressors. Because trying to conceive can be stressful, lowering stress is an effective strategy for fertility-building and preconception. Though the studied benefits of ashwagandha for fertility have mostly been focused on sperm-making, people of all genders can take ashwagandha. Enjoy it as a tincture or powder, at a dosage of 2–5 mL of tincture or 2–5 g of powder per day.

Chlorella is a microalga. While not specifically a fertility superfood, chlorella deserves a spot in the fertility-building and conception phase because of its detoxification powers. Chlorella helps protect against the effects of heavy metal exposure and pollution. Heavy metals have anti-fertility effects. They are known to disrupt hormone balance, lower semen quality, and cause genetic damage as they accumulate in the testicles.[13] From an herbal perspective, these heavy metals can be removed from the body through chelation.

Chlorella acts as a natural chelator of heavy metals—especially lead and mercury—due to its high chlorophyll content.[14] Chlorella can detoxify neurotoxins like the heavy metal mercury as well as phthalates, plasticizers, and insecticides as well as dioxins—all strong anti-fertility chemicals. Finally, chlorella is a pro-pregnancy tonic because it's rich in iron, folate, and B$_{12}$—all of which are important nutrients for conception and a healthy pregnancy. For best results, take concentrated chlorella tablets. Chlorella powder can also be added to juices and smoothies, but the strong taste and smell could be off-putting to some! Recommended dosage for chlorella tablets is 6–10 g daily.

Damiana is a mood-lifting herb with anti-anxiety benefits. It helps lift the weight of depression and hopelessness. As a nervine herb, damiana particularly benefits those who suffer from chronic stress, tension, and low mood. Damiana pairs well with nervine trophorestorative milky oats. It's an aphrodisiac that helps with getting turned on and with maintaining strong erections. In terms of fertility, damiana benefits folks dealing with infertility and the low mood and grief associated with it.

If you have an emotional reaction to the fertility drugs used during IUI and IVF, which can cause irritability and restlessness, damiana can offer help. Fertility drugs may commonly affect mood. If you doubt the impact of hormones on emotions, just think of the mood swings that happen with premenstrual syndrome (PMS) and first-trimester hormones and menopause! Because stress and depression are linked with lower pregnancy outcomes, finding support—like playing with damiana as an herbal remedy—may help lead to a higher chance of conception. You can enjoy damiana in the form of tincture, infusion, and herbal baths or soaks. Take 2–4 mL of tincture as needed, diluted in water or juice. For infusions, use 1 teaspoon of dried damiana per cup of water.

Dandelion root, like chlorella, isn't a pro-fertility herb per se. But because toxic load and exposure to environmental contaminants and pollution have been linked with low fertility, detoxifying herbs like dandelion root can assist during the pre-conception phase. Detoxifying herbs reduce the burden associated with exposure to toxins. Dandelion root is great for phthalate detox, for instance. Phthalates are known to disrupt fertility. They affect the hypothalamus-pituitary-gonadal (HPG) axis, which includes the ovaries in women and testes in men, by disrupting the binding of hormones to their receptor sites, serving as an antagonist.

Dandelion root offers strong liver protection against phthalates and other toxins, thanks to its antioxidant and anti-inflammatory activities.

What's more, dandelion root is also rich in oligosaccharides, a prebiotic that keeps your gut healthy and feeds beneficial gut bacteria. A healthy gut microbiome supports overall health, which can increase your chances of conception and pregnancy. Take dandelion root in the form of herbal teas and decoctions, syrups, tinctures, or delicious roasted dandelion root coffee. Dandelion root tincture can be taken at a dosage of 2–5 mL up to three times per day. Infusions are made with 1 tablespoon of dried root per cup of water.

Eleuthero (also called Siberian ginseng) is an adaptogen and tonic. It increases endurance, stamina, and focus. Eleuthero enhances sperm count and encourages strong erections while also supporting the health of the body as a whole. On the adaptogen spectrum, eleuthero is a more stimulating adaptogen, so it will be useful to folks who experience low energy levels throughout their conception journeys.

Enjoyed regularly, eleuthero keeps stress and fatigue at bay. It's a good remedy for reproductive challenges like infertility and reproductive assistance. Eleuthero is not a true ginseng, but it shares some of the benefits associated with ginseng. It is less stimulating than true ginseng, which makes eleuthero a more sustainable herbal ally for long-term use and for younger people. Enjoy it in the form of capsules or tincture. In powder form, it blends well with maca as a blend you can add to smoothies and warm drinks. Take 2–4 g of powdered eleuthero, split in two daily doses, or 2–8 mL of tincture. Avoid eleuthero closer to bedtime and prioritize taking it in the morning and early afternoon.

Maca is a Peruvian herb with a long history of use as a pro-fertility agent. Maca root supports fertility by promoting ovulation. It is also a nutritious herb that enhances overall health. Maca has been shown to enhance pregnancy rates by stimulating ovulation in a study that blended maca with vitex and folate. Over a six-month period, ovulation rates increased from 10 to 42.9 percent of women.[15]

As an adaptogen, maca will benefit the psychoemotional aspects of fertility work and help relieve the stresses associated with trying to conceive. Another pro-fertility benefit of maca is for underweight folks whose low body weight might make it harder to conceive. Maca is a nutritive tonic that helps put on more weight as needed. It won't usually cause weight gain in larger bodies. Take maca daily in the form of powder, tincture, or capsules. Maca powder can be taken at a dosage of 1–5 g per day. Take tincture at a dosage of 1–3 mL, up to twice per day. Capsules are often found at a 1,000-mg concentration; take 1–3 capsules per day.

Milk thistle seed is a potent liver tonic. Cleansing the liver and keeping the liver healthy support fertility and conception in several ways. First, a healthy liver keeps hormone levels in check. Folks who experience erratic menstrual cycles ovulate at irregular times, making conception more difficult. Silymarin, a liver tonic compound in milk thistle seed, has been found to enhance fertility. It works by acting as a potent antioxidant that reverses the damages of oxidative stress on fertility.[16]

Milk thistle seed also lowers the impacts of environmental toxins on both sperm and eggs. It's a regenerative and detoxifying remedy, and it's so potent that it has even been shown to offer protection against both radiation and poisonous mushrooms. Enjoy milk thistle seed in tincture form, 5–10 mL per day diluted in water or juice.

Milky oats are a deep tonic for the nervous system. Most folks love taking milky oats regularly. You might notice that you feel less stressed out, and that your moods seem more balanced. Because relieving stress is associated with better conception rates and a higher chance of pregnancy, stress-busting herbs like milky oats become useful as daily tonics during the fertility-building phase.

Milky oats are often used in situations of depression, anxiety, and burnout. They're a helpful remedy with infertility because every cycle where you don't conceive becomes a repeated disappointment that can create an emotional feedback loop of hope followed by despair. You can take milky oats in the form of tinctures, infusions, and herbal baths or soaks. Take regularly and over long periods for best results. Take 1–5 mL of tincture up to three times daily. Infusions are made with 1 tablespoon of dried milky oats per cup of water.

Nettle is a nutritive herb, which means it's rich in highly assimilable nutrients. The sex organs and reproductive system both require a steady supply of nutrients in order to function optimally. Daily nettle tea infusions support better egg quality while ensuring proper nutritional levels overall. Nettle is an iron-rich herb, which makes it ideal for menstruating people who experience heavy bleeding during menstruation, as well as for folks with restricted diets who may not consume as much iron-rich food as a result.

Nettle leaf is best enjoyed as an infusion because water acts as a potent solvent for the vitamins and minerals it contains. Use 2 teaspoons of dried nettle per cup of water for infusions. Nettle and peppermint tea is delicious, and you can add milky oats and flavorful hibiscus to the infusion as well. Fresh nettles can also be harvested in the spring and blanched for freezing. In that way, nettle can be used as a high nutrient functional food source, used in the place of spinach in most recipes. Eat liberally. Note that I've seen some studies suggest that nettle could be anti-fertility for men and specifically lower sperm quality, so use nettle as a fertility herb for women only.

Oat straw is the stems and straw of oats. It comes from the same plant as milky oats, which are the unripe seeds of the oat plant. Oat straw is primarily a nutritive herb. It's a nutrient-rich tonic that nourishes the body. Deep nourishment enhances wellness and fertility by supporting the reproductive organs, hormone balance, and healthy cycles. When you're well nourished, you're more resilient to stress. You sleep better and have more energy.

Many nutritionists find that folks are undernourished. Nourishment has nothing to do with weight and body size. Folks of all shapes and sizes can be undernourished, and it can negatively affect their fertility. Being undernourished can be caused by a variety of factors, from the impacts of diet culture to lack of access to fresh nutritious foods, for example.

Nutritive herbs like oat straw don't replace nutritious meals, but they can help provide nutrition in a convenient, sippable way. Oat straw is most commonly enjoyed as an herbal tea. That's because water extracts the vitamins and minerals in oat straw effectively. It pairs well with nettle and can be sipped on daily. Use 1 tablespoon of dried oat straw per cup of water.

Passionflower is a calming herb with an affinity for the emotional heart. It soothes and calms and helps with irritability. It helps lower anxiety and relieve depression and pain. A 2017 study demonstrated that passionflower is effective in improving resilience and quality of life in patients suffering from nervous restlessness.[17] Daily intake of passionflower for twelve weeks resulted in a significant reduction in their symptoms, which included inner restlessness, sleep disturbances, exhaustion, fear, difficulty concentrating, sweating, nausea, trembling, and palpitations. There were no adverse effects from passionflower aside from three reports of feeling mildly tired, which makes sense because passionflower is a calming herb.

Trying to conceive can be stressful, especially when the process takes longer than you thought it would. In my experience, folks start to feel some frustration or impatience after about six to twelve months of trying without achieving a pregnancy. Nervine herbs like passionflower can do wonders for your mood. The process of assisted conception like IUI and IVF are emotional roller coasters. Passionflower, damiana, and milky oats together make a great combo for psychoemotional health, along with other complementary strategies like therapy or support groups. You can take passionflower in the form of tincture or infusion. Take 1–3 mL of tincture up to three times a day. For infusions, use 1 teaspoon of dried passionflower per cup of water.

Reishi is a medicinal mushroom and deep tonic. It's an adaptogen and promotes fertility for folks of all genders by supporting the body as a whole. Reishi has liver healing benefits that make it ideal for hormonal balance in preparation for conception. Hormone balance and reproductive wellness are linked with good liver function because the liver is responsible for regulating sex hormones.

What's more, reishi mushroom is also a potent immune tonic. Because reishi supports immune modulation, folks who live with autoimmune diseases like endometriosis, celiac disease, Hashimoto's hypothyroidism, and whose conditions affect fertility, will benefit from reishi as a daily boost. Reishi also delivers stress-relieving adaptogenic benefits during the pre-conception phase. Take reishi daily in the form of tinctures or decoctions. Tinctures can be taken at a dosage of 2–4 mL up to three times per day. For decoctions, use 3–5 slices of dried reishi per 4 cups of water, and drink 1–2 cups daily.

Schisandra berry is a remedy from Traditional Chinese Medicine (TCM), just like reishi. It's a pro-fertility adaptogen. Schisandra berry is a balancing, stress-relieving herb that supports the reproductive organs and healthy cycles. One of the benefits of schisandra berry is its effect on hormones and liver health. It is a hepatic trophorestorative, which means it works as a liver tonic. A healthy liver paves the way for balanced hormones and cycles.

It's an herbal ally during the fertility-building and pre-conception phase as well as during assisted conception like IUI or IVF. Schisandra also works well as an aphrodisiac because it relieves stress and provides stable energy levels. Enjoy schisandra berry in the form of decoctions, syrups, tinctures, or powder. For decoctions, use 1 tablespoon of dried berries per cup of water. Drink one cup daily. Tincture can be taken at a dosage of 1–3 mL up to three times daily. Schisandra powder can be taken at a dosage of 1–3 g per day, with meals.

Shatavari is a traditional herb of Ayurveda. It is considered to be a therapeutic female tonic for reproductive wellness. Shatavari increases egg quality and follicular growth and development by reducing the oxidative stress load in the body.[18] Shatavari also increases vaginal lubrication, which supports conception because it provides a welcoming environment for sperm to travel to the uterus. As an adaptogen, shatavari root helps women balance their hormones and reduce the stress load associated with low fertility and PCOS.

Adaptogenic benefits are helpful to folks who are fertility-building and trying to conceive. That's because adaptogens help your body be more resilient to various stressors, all while supporting healthy moods and energy levels. Shatavari can be taken in tincture form, capsules, or as a powder added to drinks and plant lattes. As a tincture, take 1–3 mL up to three times daily. Shatavari powder can be taken at a dosage of up to 5 g. It also makes delicious bliss balls when shatavari powder is blended with nut butter and honey, and can be paired with maca for the purpose of fertility-building.

Turmeric is a general tonic. As an antioxidant, turmeric root reverses the anti-fertility damage of oxidative stress, which is an excess of free radicals in the body. The best way to enjoy turmeric during the pre-conception phase is to consume it in small doses as a healing food. Avoid supplements, which can be too concentrated. Note that therapeutic doses of turmeric and curcumin could negatively affect women's fertility, so use it mostly with male bodies for that purpose. The way turmeric could lower women's fertility has to do with uterine lining thickness—high doses of turmeric could presumably thin it and make implantation less likely. That being said, small doses of whole turmeric powder or fresh turmeric rhizome used in cooking—like in curries— are safe. Used as a food, turmeric could promote fertility for all genders by acting as a general tonic and liver tonic. Use turmeric root in powder form, added to warm drinks and foods, about 1–3 g per day.

Vitex is widely known as a reproductive tonic for women's bodies. That's because it has progesterone-type activity within the body, which means it can improve menstrual regularity for people who have low progesterone or a too-short luteal phase. In other words, vitex balances estrogen and progesterone release throughout the menstrual cycle. This in turn improves chances of conception.

Vitex can assist with symptoms of PMS and premenstrual dysphoric disorder (PMDD) while enhancing fertility levels in folks with menstrual disorders. Take vitex in the form of capsules or tincture, at a dosage of 200 mg per day or 1–3 mL of tincture up to three times per day. Vitex isn't a general tonic and shouldn't be consumed daily for long periods. Vitex isn't for everyone; consult with an herbalist for best results.